Published By Nicholas Thompson

@ Herbert Cox

Low Fodmap Diet: Easy and Healthy Low-fodmap

Recipes to With Delicious and Nutritious Diet

All Right RESERVED

ISBN 978-1-7782903-2-9

TABLE OF CONTENTS

Spiced Quinoa With Almonds & Feta

Ingredients:

- 50g toasted flaked almonds

- 100g feta cheese , crumbled

- Handful parsley , roughly chopped

- Juice ½ lemon

- 1 tbsp olive oil

- 1 tsp ground coriander

- ½ tsp turmeric

- 300g quinoa , rinsed

Directions:

1. Heat the oil in a large pan. Add the spices, then fry for a min or so until fragrant.

2. Add the quinoa, then fry for a further min until you can hear gentle popping sounds.

3. Stir in 600ml boiling water, then gently simmer for 10-15 mins until the water has evaporated and the quinoa grains have a white 'halo' around them.
4. Allow to cool slightly, then stir through the other ingredients.
5. Serve warm or cold.

Roast Sea Bass & Vegetable Traybake

Ingredients:

- 1 rosemary sprig, leaves removed and very finely chopped

- 2 sea bass fillets

- 25g pitted black olive, halved

- ½ lemon, sliced thinly into rounds

- 300g red-skinned potatoes, thinly sliced into rounds

- 1 red pepper, cut into strips

- 2 tbsp extra virgin olive oil

- Handful basil leaves

Directions:

1. Heat oven to 180C/160C fan/gas 4.

2. Arrange the potato and pepper slices on a large non-stick baking tray.

3. Drizzle over 1 tbsp oil and scatter with the rosemary, a pinch of salt and a good grinding of pepper.

4. Toss everything together well and roast for 25 mins, turning over halfway through, until the potatoes are golden and crisp at the edges.

5. Arrange the fish fillets on top and scatter over the olives.

6. Place a couple of lemon slices on top of the fish and drizzle with the remaining oil.

7. Roast for further 7-8 mins until the fish is cooked through. Serve scattered with basil leaves.

Roasted Ratatouille Vegetable Enchiladas With Fire Roasted Tomato Sauce

Ingredients:

- 1 large eggplant cut into ½ inch cubes

- 1 medium zucchini 1/2 pound, cut into ½ inch cubes

- 1 medium patty pan or summer squash cut into ½ inch cubes

- 1 red bell pepper diced

- 1 cup chicken or vegetable stock

- 2 tablespoons fresh lime juice

- 2/3 cup coarsely grated cheddar cheese

- Eight 6-inch corn or almond flour tortillas

- ½ cup cilantro leaves

- 2 pounds vine or Roma tomatoes quartered

- 1 jalapeno halved (ribs and seeds optional)

- ½ teaspoon ground cumin

- ½ teaspoon ground coriander

- Olive oil

- Sea salt

Directions:

1. Preheat your oven to 425°F. Line two sheet pans with parchment paper.

2. Place the tomatoes and the jalapeño on one of the sheet pans. Drizzle with olive oil and season with the cumin, coriander and ½ teaspoon salt. Arrange cut-side down and roast in the oven until slightly charred, about 40 minutes.

3. On the second sheet pan, toss the eggplant, zucchini and peppers with 2 tablespoons olive

oil and ½ teaspoon salt. Arrange in an even layer and roast alongside the tomatoes in the oven for about 45 minutes, until nicely caramelized. Set aside to cool.

4. Transfer the tomatoes and jalapeño to a blender or food processor and add any cooking juices from the sheet pan, along with the stock, lime juice and ½-teaspoon salt. Process until smooth. You should have about 3 cups sauce.

5. In a large mixing bowl, toss the ratatouille filling with a third of the sauce and 1/3 cup of cheese.

6. Pour another third of the tomato sauce in the bottom of a 9-by-13-inch baking dish. Spread the sauce to cover the bottom.

7. Wrap the tortillas in a dishtowel and warm them in the microwave for 30 seconds until pliable. Alternatively, you can warm them in the oven.

8. Divide the veggies evenly among the tortillas. Roll up the tortillas tightly around the ratatouille and line them up, seam-side down, in the baking dish. Pour the remaining tomato sauce evenly over the stuffed tortillas and sprinkle with the remaining cheese.

9. Bake the enchiladas until the cheese is melted and golden brown and the sauce is bubbling, about 20 minutes. Sprinkle with the cilantro and serve immediately.

Eggplant-Kale Caponata Lasagna

Ingredients:

- 2 cups low FODMAP tomato sauce 16 ounces

- 2 tablespoons golden raisins

- 1 tablespoon balsamic vinegar

- ¼ cup torn basil leaves divided

- 9 ounces gluten-free no boil lasagna noodles about 6 sheets

- 8 ounces plant-based ricotta optional

- 5 ounces shredded mozzarella I used a combo of part-skim and fresh mozz

- 2 tablespoons olive oil

- 1 medium eggplant 3/4 pound, diced

- 1/2 teaspoon sea salt

- ½ teaspoon red chili flakes

- 1 medium vine or Roma tomato diced

- 8 ounces frozen chopped kale or 1 bunch finely chopped

Directions:

1. Preheat the oven to 350 degrees.
2. In a large skillet, heat the olive oil. Sauté the eggplant over medium-high heat until beginning to soften, about 8 minutes. Add the salt and red pepper flakes. Stir in the tomatoes, scrapping up any brown bits from the bottom of the pan. Sauté until the tomatoes have softened, about 3 minutes. Add the kale and continue to sauté until very wilted and the liquid has evaporated, about 4 minutes more.
3. Remove from the heat and add the raisins, balsamic and half the basil.

4. Spread 1/2 cup of the tomato sauce in the bottom of a 9 x 13 casserole dish. Arrange your first layer of noodles on top, making sure they overlap slightly. Slather the noodles with half the ricotta, if using, followed by half the eggplant mixture, followed by another 1/2 cup sauce and ¼ cup mozzarella. Repeat the layers once more.

5. Finish the lasagna with a final layer of noodles, tomato sauce, the remaining cheese and basil leaves.

6. Bake in the oven for 30-40 minutes, or until the noodles are tender and the top of the lasagna is beginning to brown.

7. Allow the lasagna to rest for 5 minutes before cutting it into slabs and serving.

Winter Salad With Spaghetti Squash, Lentil + Arugula

Ingredients:

- 1/4 cup feta cheese crumbles

- Lemon tahini dressing:

- 2 tablespoons tahini

- 1 1/2 tablespoons fresh squeezed lemon juice

- 1/2 tablespoon garlic infused oil

- 1/2 tablespoon water

- 1 cup cooked spaghetti squash (about 1/2 small squash)

- 1 cup canned lentils (drained and rinsed) or 1/2 cup cooked green lentils

- 1 medium carrot, sliced

- 2 cups fresh arugula

- 1/3 cup pomegranate arils

- Salt and pepper, to taste

Directions:

1. Layer salad ingredients: squash, lentils, carrot slices, arugula, pomegranate arils then feta on small platter.
2. Whisk together lemon tahini dressing ingredients.
3. Drizzle dressing over salad.

Salad With Marinated "Feta- Style" Tofu

Ingredients:

- Dash of red pepper flakes, optional

- Salt and pepper, to taste

- 4 cup lettuce greens

- 20 cherry tomatoes, cut in half

- 20 green beans, trimmed, raw

- 1 red bell pepper, de-seeded, cut in strips

- 1/4 cup pitted kalamata olives

- 400 g firm tofu

- 2 lemons

- 2 tablespoons white miso

- 1 tablespoon oregano (dried)

- 1/4 cup garlic infused olive oil

- 1 tablespoon nutritional yeast (optional)

- 1 tablespoon apple cider vinegar

- 3 tablespoons water

Directions:

1. Press excess water out of tofu by placing tofu on a plate, in between two paper towels and place something heavy on top. Leave in place for about 30 minutes.

2. Meanwhile, prepare marinade in medium bowl, add juice of one lemon, miso, oregano, 2 tablespoons garlic infused olive oil, nutritional yeast, if using, apple cider vinegar, water, red pepper flakes, if using and salt and pepper, to taste. Whisk mixture with a whisk or fork until blended.

3. Cut firm tofu, into bite size pieces. Add tofu to bowl with marinade. Gently stir tofu, covering in marinade. Cover bowl with plastic wrap and

place in the refrigerator to marinate for about 1-2 hours.

4. Prepare salad by arranging lettuce, cherry tomatoes, raw green beans, red bell pepper slices and olives. Top with marinated "feta-style" tofu on top. (you can save some extra tofu and use for another dish, or top it all on the salad. Just keep your portion at around 2/3 cup of firm tofu per serving)

5. Dress salad with remaining lemon (cut and drizzle lemon juice) and garlic infused oil, over vegetables, along with salt and pepper, if desired.

Fish Stew

Ingredients:

- 500 grams of mussels, cleaned, with the facial hair

- eliminated 200 ml of water

- Pinch of salt

- Pinch of newly broke dark pepper

- Handful of basil and level leaf parsley, generally chopped

- 3 tablespoons of garlic-injected olive

- oil 200 grams of cubed pancetta

- 2 teaspoons of paprika

- 1 piece of red bean stew, seeds eliminated and hacked finely 500 ml of dry white wine

- 500 grams of cod filets, skins and bones eliminated 6 ready enormous tomatoes, cut into chunks

Directions:

1. Place a huge skillet on the oven over medium hotness settings. Place 2 tablespoons of garlic-implanted olive oil and hotness slightly.
2. Add the pancetta shapes and cook until sautéed, around 2-3 minutes.
3. Add stew and paprika. Give a speedy stir. Add white wine.
4. Bring this to a bubble then, at that point, lessen the hotness to a stew.
5. Permit the combination to stew for a couple minutes.
6. Add the cod filets, trailed by the cut tomatoes.
7. Place the mussels last.
8. Add water and season with salt and pepper.

9. Cover and stew for 10 minutes.

10. Turn off the hotness and eliminate the cover.

11. Dispose of any mussels that poor person opened.

12. Sprinkle the new spices. Take the excess 1 tablespoon of olive oil and sprinkle over the soup. Serve warm in bowls.

Mulligatawny Soup

Ingredients:

- 1 enormous potato, eliminate the strip and cut into 2.5 cm

- 3D shapes 700 grams courgette, unpeeled and cut into

- 2.5cm blocks 225 grams of tomatoes, skin stripped and chopped

- 75 grams of basmati rice

- 850 ml of water

- 1 teaspoon of fennel seeds

- 1 teaspoon of cumin seeds

- 1 teaspoon of coriander seeds

- Seeds from 3 entire cases of cardamom 2 tablespoons of olive oil

- Salt and pepper, for preparing

- Handful of chives, cleaved finely

Directions:

1. Place a huge pot over medium high hotness.

2. Place the flavors (cardamom seeds, coriander seeds, fennel seeds, cumin seeds) and softly toast until fragrant.

3. Remove from the pan and move to a mortar.

4. Ground into a fine powder with a pestle. Set aside.

5. In a similar pan, add olive oil. Heat a little then, at that point, add courgette, tomatoes and potatoes.

6. Season with pepper and a touch of salt.

7. Add the powdered flavors. Sauté for a couple minutes.

8. Add water and permit to stew for 20 minutes.

9. In the event that the vegetables turn delicate, they're now cooked.

10. Eliminate the pan from the hotness and put away to cool slightly.

11. Once somewhat cooled, place half of the vegetables in a blender or food processor. Beat until smooth.

12. Bring 175 ml of water to a bubble in a different pot.

13. Add basmati rice and diminish the hotness to a low stew.

14. Cook for 10-15 minutes until rice becomes tender.

15. Return the mixed portion of the soup to the pot.

16. Blend well in with the remainder of the vegetables.

17. Remove the cooked rice from the pot and add to the vegetables.

18. Mix to circulate the rice well all through the soup.

19. Serve finished off with hacked chives.

Banana Pancakes

Ingredients:

- 2 tbsp of gluten-free all-purpose flour

- 3 tbsp of olive oil spread OR dairy-free butter

- Powdered sugar

- ¼ tsp of baking powder

- ½ tsp of ground cinnamon

- ¼ tsp of ground nutmeg

- 1 pinch of salt

- 1 large mixing bowl

- 1 large frying pan

- 2 firm bananas

- 10 blueberries

- 2 large eggs

- 6 tbsp of lactose-free yogurt (or coconut yogurt)

- 1 tbsp of brown sugar (tightly packed)

Directions:

1. Begin by peeling the bananas and mashing them in a large mixing bowl.
2. Add in the eggs and whisk in the bananas.
3. Combine the salt, cinnamon, gluten-free flour, nutmeg, brown sugar, and baking powder with the bananas, and make sure to mix well.
4. Add a tablespoon of your dairy-free spread to a frying pan as it heats up on a medium flame.
5. Start cooking the pancakes by scooping about 3 tbsp of batter into the pan, one at a time.
6. Once you see bubbles beginning to form on the top surface of the pancake, flip and allow it to cook until both sides are golden brown.

7. Continue cooking the pancakes until you are out of batter on consistent heat and adding more dairy-free spread if necessary.
8. Serve the pancakes in a stack with your yogurt and berries.
9. Sprinkle powdered sugar on top of the pancakes if you desire. Enjoy!

Green Smoothie

Ingredients:

- 1 whole kiwi

- 1-2 2 cups of ice cubes

- 2 cups of baby spinach (you can use Lacinato Kale leaves for a more intense flavor)

- 1 blender or food processor

- Approx. 8 inches of an English cucumber

- 1 cup of green grapes (try for seedless grapes)

Directions:

1. Begin by figuring out which end of your blender the blade is on.
2. We want to put the grapes either first or last, depending on the blade position so that they get the blending process started smoothly.

3. Next, peel your kiwi and cut it into large chunks. Leave the English cucumber unpeeled, and cut that into chunks as well, a little smaller this time.

4. If you are using kale leaves rather than baby spinach, make sure the kale is properly washed, stemmed, and roughly chopped.

5. Now, add all your INGREDIENTS:, except the ice cubes, to the blender, making sure to keep the grapes closest to the blade.

6. Pulse your blender on and off a few times to get the INGREDIENTS: to blend slightly, and then blend at high speed until you see a green, homogeneous mixture in your blender.

7. There should be no chunks or pieces of grated leaves in there.

8. Once the mixture is ready, add a few ice cubes at a time and blend everything together until the smoothie becomes a little frosty.

9. You can continue adding ice if you desire. It will help thicken the smoothie and cool your drink.

10. Pour into a glass and drink before the INGREDIENTS: begin to separate. Enjoy!

11. In this recipe, we used grapes and kiwi because they can offer either sweet or tangy flavors, depending on how ripe they are.

12. Since the ripeness does not change the FODMAP count in either fruit, you are at liberty to choose how ripe you would like your fruits to be, particularly kiwi.

13. We also recommend that first-time green smoothie drinkers use baby spinach instead of kale.

14. Spinach has a much milder flavor, whereas kale offers a bold flavor that some people can find overwhelming if they are not used to it.

15. Finally, feel free to add in a handful of low-FODMAP berries into this smoothie as long as

you stay within the recommended FODMAP serving sizes.

16. Enjoy your customizable smoothie!

Deviled Eggs

Ingredients:

- 1/8 teaspoon salt

- 1/8 teaspoon pepper

- 12 black olives

- 6 hard-boiled eggs, halved

- 3 tablespoons mayonnaise

- 1 teaspoon Dijon mustard

- 1 teaspoon vinegar

Directions:

1. Cut eggs in half lengthwise.
2. Using a spoon, remove the yolk from the whites, being careful not to ruin the shape of the whites.

3. Mash the yolks with a fork, stirring in the chopped black olives, the mayonnaise, mustard, vinegar, salt and pepper.
4. Place the yolks back into the eggs with your spoon or a decorative piping tool.
5. Sprinkle with paprika and serve.

Eggs And Fries

Ingredients:

- 1 tsp smoked paprika

- 2 tomatoes, halved

- 2 eggs

- 2 medium baking potatoes, cut into chunky wedges

- 2 T olive oil

Directions:

1. Heat the oven to 375F. Place the potato wedges into a 9 x 13 baking pan.
2. Drizzle the olive oil over the potatoes, stirring to thoroughly coat them.
3. Sprinkle the paprika over the potatoes and stir again.

4. Place in the oven for 25 minutes, partially roasting the potatoes.
5. Pull the potatoes and flip them all with a spatula.
6. Place the tomatoes, cut side to the upside, in between the potatoes, like a kind of nest.
7. Scooch out the potatoes to allow for space for the two eggs, and crack an egg into each space.
8. Place back in the oven and cook for 68 minutes until the potatoes and eggs are done to your liking.

Breakfast Muesli

Ingredients:

- 7 tablespoons olive oil

- 8 tablespoons dried coconut, shredded

- 65 grams brown sugar

- 5 tablespoons pumpkin seeds

- 250 grams low FODMAP cornflakes, gluten-free

- 30 grams banana chips, dried

- 38 grams quinoa puffs

Directions:

1. Set the oven to 150 degrees Celsius.
2. Crush the cornflakes roughly and place them in a large bowl together with pumpkin seeds, quinoa puffs, brown sugar and coconut. Cover the mixture with oil.

3. Spread the mixture evenly on a roasting tray that is lined with baking paper.
4. Toast the muesli in the oven for about 20 minutes. Remember to shake the tray halfway through the cook.
5. Once the muesli is light brown in color, remove the tray from the oven and set aside to cool.
6. Crush the banana chips lightly and add it to the mixture.

Rhubarb Custard Cups

Ingredients:

- 2 teaspoons vanilla extract

- 5 tablespoons custard powder

- 1 ½ teaspoons white sugar

- 1 liter almond milk

- 300 grams fresh rhubarb, chopped

- 3 cups muesli

- 40 grams fresh raspberries

Directions:

1. Put the strawberries and rhubarb in a saucepan.
2. Add enough amount of water to cover the fruits completely.
3. Allow the mixture to simmer over medium heat for about 10 minutes.

4. Once the rhubarb has turned soft, remove the
    excess liquid from the mixture using a sieve
    and place it back in the saucepan. Mash the
    stewed fruits.

5. To make your own custard, mix the remaining
    INGREDIENTS: together in a large bowl until a
    smooth consistency is obtained.

6. Place the custard mixture in the microwave
    and cook it on high for 2 minutes.

7. Give the mixture a stir and heat it in the
    microwave for another 2 minutes.

8. Do this repeatedly until the custard becomes
    thick.

9. Spread the custard evenly at the bottom of
    the cup.

10. Place a layer of muesli on top followed by the
    stewed rhubarb. Repeat the process until cups
    are almost full.

Baked Eggs With Spinach Plus Labneh

Ingredients:

- 50 g child spinach leaves.

- 4 eggs.

- 2 tablespoons labneh (goat's cheddar or feta additionally function admirably).

- 4 sprigs of dill.

- 1 teaspoon coconut oil, in addition to extra for lubing.

- 200 g tinned Roma tomatoes, generally hacked.

- 2 bunch cherry tomatoes split.

Directions:

1. Preheat the stove to 200°C/400°F/Gas Mark 6.

2. Warm a little griddle over medium warmth and soften the coconut oil in it.

3. Include the entirety of the tomatoes and cook for 2 minutes, at that point expel from the warmth.

4. Softly oil four 250 ml (9 fl oz/1 cup) limit ramekins with coconut oil.

5. Partition the child spinach and sautéed tomatoes equitably between the ramekins, at that point break an egg into each home of spinach and tomatoes.

6. Spot a dab of labneh over each egg and top with a sprig of dill, at that point place the ramekins on a preparing plate (heating sheet) and prepare in the broiler for 18 minutes.

7. When cooked, expel from the broiler and let represent 5 minutes before serving.

Potato & Egg Salad

Ingredients:

- 1 little cucumber

- 3 tbsp new chives

- 3 tbsp green onions/scallions (green tips only)

- 85 ml (1/3 cup) mayonnaise

- 1 tbsp lemon juice

- 1 tbsp wholegrain mustard

- 800 g potato

- 160 g green beans

- 4 huge egg

- 1 red chili peppers

- Season with dark pepper

Directions:

1. Scour and cut the potatoes into reduced down pieces (strip if vital).

2. Set up the green beans by cutting into little pieces.

3. Spot the potatoes in an enormous pan and cover with water.

4. Spot the cover on the pot and carry the water to a turning bubble over medium-high warmth.

5. At that point turn down the heat to medium-low and permit to bubble for 15 to 20 minutes until the potatoes are delicate.

6. Add the green beans to the pot, around 3 minutes before you channel the potatoes.

7. Enable the green beans to cook for 2 to 3 minutes, until delicate and brilliantly shaded. Deplete and spot to the other side to cool.

8. While the potatoes cook, hard-heat up the eggs.

9. Spot the eggs in a little pot of water and spread with cold water. Spot the pan over medium-high warmth and carry the water to a moving bubble.

10. Permit to bubble for two minutes before turning the heat down to the least warmth setting.

11. Cook for 10 to 12 minutes. Deplete and run the eggs under cold water before stripping. Cut the eggs into quarters.

12. While the eggs cook, set up the cucumber and red chili peppers.

13. Strip the cucumber and cut into off sticks.

14. Deseed and bones the red ringer peppers. Finely hack the green onions/scallions (green tips just) and chives.

15. Make the plate of mixed greens dressing by combining the wholegrain mustard, mayonnaise, lemon juice and two or three toils of dark pepper.

16. In an enormous bowl delicately combine the potatoes, green beans, hard-bubbled eggs, cucumber, red chime peppers, green onions/scallions (green tips just), chives and plate of mixed greens dressing.

17. Season with a few drudgeries of dark pepper.

18. Enjoy yourself

Pasta Carbonara

Ingredients:

- 15 g butter

- 1 tablespoon of grated Parmesan

- 160 g of gluten-free penne 60 g bacon, diced

- 1 egg Salt Pepper

Directions:

1. Cook the pasta in boiling salted water.
2. Brown the bacon in a non-stick pan. Once cooked, place it on absorbent paper to remove some of the fat.
3. Break the eggs into a bowl, with a pinch of salt and pepper, and beat them well with a fork.
4. Drain the pasta and pour it into the bowl. Stir quickly to cook the eggs in contact with the pasta.

5. Add the bacon, butter and Parmesan grated. Finally serve.

Spaghetti With Citrus Pesto

Ingredients:

- 4 anchovy fillets (optional)

- ½ tablespoon of lemon juice

- ½ tablespoon of maple syrup

- 2 tablespoons of extra virgin olive oil

- 160 g of gluten-free spaghetti

- 5 basil leaves

- ½ orange

- 23 g of almonds

- 25 g of capers

- Salt

Directions:

1. Wash and dry the basil leaves or, if they are not dirty, gently clean them with a damp cloth and dab them between 2 sheets of absorbent paper.

2. Peel the orange, remove the white filaments and put it in the blender together with the almonds, capers, anchovies (optional), basil, lemon juice and maple syrup.

3. Blend until you get a homogeneous mixture. Finally slowly add the oil and continue to blend until creamy.

4. Put the pesto in a bowl and cover with a drizzle of oil to prevent oxidation.

5. Close tightly with a lid or cling film. Keep refrigerated until consumed.

6. While cooking the spaghetti, transfer the citrus pesto to a bowl and add 4 or 5 tablespoons of the pasta cooking water.

7. Drain the spaghetti and put them back in the cooking pot. Season with the pesto, mix well and serve.

Tomato Tostadas

Ingredients:

- 1 tsp of dry parsley

- ¼ tsp of ground black pepper

- 2 tbsp of fresh lemon juice

- 1 tbsp of brown sugar

- 1 tbsp of dry oregano

- 3 tbsp of olive oil

- 4 gluten-free tortillas

- 1 cup of cherry tomatoes, cut in half

- 1 cup of red cabbage, finely chopped

- 2 pieces of chicken breast, shredded into large pieces

- 1 tbsp of chili sauce, gluten-free

- 1 cup of lactose-free sour cream

- ½ tsp of salt

- 1 tsp of ground garlic

Directions:

1. Heat up the olive oil over medium-high temperature. First you want to fry tortillas, one at a time.

2. They should be golden and crispy. This process will take 3-4 minutes for each tortilla. Soak the excess oil with kitchen paper.

3. Combine the tomatoes and oregano and add to the saucepan. Stir well and fry for 2-3 minutes, over a medium temperature. Season with salt and pepper.

4. Add garlic, parsley, lemon juice. Stir well, reduce the heat to minimum and add chicken.

5. Fry for about 30 minutes, stir occasionally.

6. Remove from the heat when the meat softens and gets nice golden color.

7. In a bowl, whisk together cabbage, lactose-free sour cream, gluten-free chili sauce and sugar.

8. You want a smooth and creamy mixture.

9. Top each tortilla with chicken mixture and cream dressing. Serve warm.

Roasted Avocado

Ingredients:

- 3 eggs

- 3 tbsp of olive oil

- 2 tsp of dried rosemary

- 3 medium ripe avocados, cut in half

- Salt and pepper to taste

Directions:

1. Preheat oven to 350 degrees.
2. Cut avocado in half and remove the flesh from the center.
3. Place one egg in each avocado half and sprinkle with rosemary, salt and pepper.
4. Grease the baking pan with olive oil and place the avocados.

5. You want to use a small baking pan so your avocados can fit tightly. Place in the oven for about 15-20 minutes.

Oven-Baked Egg & Chips

Ingredients:

- 1 tsp smoked paprika

- 2 tomatoes , halved

- 2 eggs

- 2 medium baking potatoes , cut into chunky wedges

- 2 tbsp olive oil

Directions:

1. Heat oven to 190C/170C fan/gas 5. Tip the potato wedges into a roasting tin.
2. Drizzle over the oil and sprinkle over the paprika.
3. Season and mix well to coat the potatoes.
4. Roast for 25 mins, turning halfway through, until almost tender.

5. Nestle the tomatoes, cut-side up, amongst the potatoes.

6. Make 2 spaces in the tin and crack an egg into each one. Return to the oven for 6-8 mins until the eggs are just set.

Egg & New Potato Salad

Ingredients:

- Handful chopped parsley

- Hard boiled egg

- Bag of wild rocket

- Cucumber , diced, to serve

- Hot boiled new potatoes

- 2 tbsp olive oil

- Juice of 1/2 lemon

Directions:

1. Toss some hot boiled new potatoes with the olive oil, lemon juice and parsley.
2. Leave to cool, then toss with quartered hard-boiled eggs.

3. Toss with wild rocket leaves and some diced
    cucumber to serve.

Healthy Fish & Chips With Tartare Sauce

Ingredients:

- 1 tbsp capers , chopped

- 2 heaped tbsp 0% greek yogurt

- Lemon wedge, to serve

- 450g potatoes , peeled and cut into chips

- 1 tbsp olive oil , plus a little extra for brushing

- 2 white fish fillets about 140g/5oz each

- Grated zest and juice 1 lemon

- Small handful of parsley leaves, chopped

Directions:

1. Heat oven to 200C/fan 180C/gas 6. Toss chips in oil.
2. Spread over a baking sheet in an even layer, bake for 40 mins until browned and crisp.
3. Put the fish in a shallow dish, brush lightly with oil, salt and pepper.
4. Sprinkle with half the lemon juice, bake for 12-15 mins.
5. After 10 mins sprinkle over a little parsley and lemon zest to finish cooking.
6. Meanwhile, mix the capers, yogurt, remaining parsley and lemon juice together, set aside and season if you wish.
7. To serve, divide the chips between plates, lift the fish onto the plates and serve with a spoonful of yogurt mix.

Tamari-Balsamic Steak And Grilled Vegetable Marinade

Ingredients:

- 1 tablespoon honey or maple syrup

- ½ teaspoon salt

- 1 minced garlic clove optional

- ¼ cup balsamic or red wine vinegar

- ¼ cup Dijon mustard

- ¼ cup tamari or gluten-free soy sauce

- ¼ olive oil

Directions:

1. In a small mixing bowl or 2-cup measure, whisk together the vinegar, Dijon and tamari.

2. Slowly whisk in the olive oil until it emulsifies and incorporates easily. Sweeten with the

honey or maple syrup, and season with the salt. Stir in the garlic if using.

3. To use with grilled vegetables: brush both sides of your vegetables (zucchini, squash, Portobello mushrooms, eggplant, etc.) or vegetable kabobs with the marinade and season with salt. Grill over medium-high heat on both sides, rotating 90 degrees halfway through to get a nice cross-hatch, until nicely charred.

4. To use with roasted vegetables: Preheat the oven to 425 degrees.

5. Toss 1 pound of chopped vegetables (cauliflower, broccoli, asparagus, mushrooms, etc.) with ¼ cup of marinade.

6. Arrange in an even layer and season lightly with salt. Roast until lightly browned, about 20 minutes depending on the vegetable.

7. To use with steak: Marinate 1 pound of steak (we like rib eye, flank steak, skirt steak or

fillet) for 30 minutes in ½ cup of marinade. Remove the meat from the marinade and season generously with salt and pepper.

8. Sear over high heat on the stovetop or grill until medium rare and nicely charred on both sides.

Gluten-Free Bruschetta Pasta Salad

Ingredients:

- 1 teaspoon sea salt

- 1 cup basil leaves finely chopped

- 12 ounces gluten-free pasta

- 1 1/2 pounds mixed tomatoes finely diced

- 1 small garlic clove minced

- 1 tablespoon balsamic vinegar

- ¼ cup extra virgin olive oil

- ½ teaspoon red pepper flakes

Directions:

1. In a large mixing bowl, combine the tomatoes, garlic, balsamic, olive oil, red pepper flakes, salt, and half the basil.

2. Allow to sit for up to an hour at room temperature or longer in the fridge so the tomatoes have time to marinate and absorb the entire added flavor.

3. Bring a large pot of salted water to boil over high heat.

4. Cook the pasta according to package directions until al dente.

5. Drain and add to the bowl with the tomato mixture.

6. Toss the hot pasta with the tomatoes. Taste for seasoning and add the remaining basil right before serving.

Cream Puff Cake

Ingredients:

Cake:

- 1 cup gluten free flour blend

- 4 large eggs, at room temperature

- 1 cup water

- 1/2 cup butter

Cream filling:

- 2 tablespoons confectioner's sugar

- 1/2 teaspoon vanilla

- 1 cup whipping cream

Directions:

1. Preheat oven to 400 degrees F.
2. Line large baking sheet with parchment paper.

3. In medium sauce pan, bring water and butter to boil. Add the flour and stir quickly until the mixture becomes a well mixed ball of dough.

4. Add in one egg at a time, blending until the dough is smooth.

5. Drop dough onto baking sheet in 10 large rounded balls that touch each other in the shape of a wreath.

6. Bake cake for 40 minutes or until puffs are risen and bottom of cake is lightly browned.

7. Cool cake and whip up whipped cream filling.

8. In cooled metal or glass bowl, (chill in the refrigerator for about 20 minutes), add whipping cream, confectioner's sugar and vanilla. Beat with electric beaters on medium high until whipped cream is formed.

9. Carefully, slice cake in half horizontally- (if any of the cake top breaks apart, don't worry, as you will be placing it on top of the whipped cream which acts like "glue".)

10. Layer whipped cream on bottom half of cake then add back cake top.

11. Drizzle the warmed hot fudge sauce on top of the cake and let set in refrigerator. Alternatively, refrigerate cake without fudge sauce and sprinkle with confectioner's sugar right before serving.

Prosciutto Carbonara With Kale

Ingredients:

- 12 ounces suitable gluten free pasta

- 1 cup sliced kale, stems removed or use baby kale

- Garnish and season with salt, pepper, crushed red pepper flakes, as desired.

- 2 tablespoons extra virgin olive oil

- 3 ounces prosciutto, sliced in bite size strips

- 2 large eggs, plus 2 egg yolks

- 1/4 cup Parmesan or Romano cheese, grated

Directions:

1. Boil past per package directions-minus 1 minute of the suggested cooking time.

2. As pasta is cooking, add 1 tablespoon olive oil into large skillet over medium heat with prosciutto to lightly brown up, remove from heat.
3. Remove proscuitto onto plate.
4. When pasta is done, save about 1 cup of the pasta water and strain pasta.
5. Add eggs and yolks to small bowl, add cheese, 1/4 cup warm pasta water and whisk together.
6. Add remaining oil to large skillet, put heat on low.
7. Add pasta and egg mixture to skillet. Stir to blend. Add the remaining pasta water until you create a light 'sauce'.
8. Add kale to just cook lightly so it is tender but still bright green.
9. Add prosciutto and fold in to blend.
10. Garnish as desired!

Chicken Noodle Soup

Ingredients:

- 1-inch piece of entire ginger

- 1 sound leaf

- 1 medium-sized carrot, cut into short and
  slender sticks

- 80 grams of fine dried rice noodles, break into
  more limited pieces Handful of new chives,
  cleaved finely

- 4 chicken drumsticks, skin removed

- 1.2 liters of water, heat to the
  point of boiling

- 2 tablespoons of soy sauce

- Pepper and salt for seasoning

Directions:

1. In a medium-sized pot, place the drumsticks, cove leaf, ginger and soy sauce.
2. Add water and spot over medium high hotness.
3. Heat to the point of boiling, cover the pot and diminish the hotness down to a stew.
4. Allow the soup to stew on low for 40 minutes.
5. Take out chicken drumsticks, ginger and inlet leaf.
6. Add cleaved carrots to the saucepan.
7. Remove the meat from the bones.
8. Place chicken meat back into the saucepan. Add rice noodles.
9. Cover and cook for 4 additional minutes.
10. Remove the cover and sprinkle the cleaved chives. Really take a look at the taste and change flavors (pepper and salt).

Baked Fish

Ingredients:

- 4 haddock filets, skins eliminated (can substitute other sort of white fish)

- 2 tablespoons of garlic imbued olive oil

- Juice from 1 lemon

- Pinch of pepper and salt, as wanted for seasoning

- 750 grams of child potatoes

- 250 grams of cherry tomatoes, still on the plant 70 grams of pitted dark olives

- Large modest bunch of basil leaves, new and slashed roughly

Directions:

1. Preheat broiler to gas 6, 200˚C or 400˚F.

2. In a pot, heat up the child potatoes for around 15 minutes or until recently cooked. Channel the water.

3. Get a huge baking plate and put the child potatoes.

4. Add the olives and the tomatoes (counting the plant).

5. Set haddock filets on top of the vegetables.

6. Drizzle garlic-mixed olive oil all around the fish and the vegetables.

7. Pour or press the lemon juice over the fish and vegetables. Season as per taste with salt and pepper.

8. Cover the baking plate with aluminum foil.

9. Cook in the broiler for 15 minutes. Make sure that the fish is cooked well.

10. Eliminate from the broiler and top with basil leaves before serving.

Lemongrass And Coconut Chicken

Ingredients:

- 2 stalks of lemongrass, cleaved roughly

- 30 grams of creamed coconut, slashed around

- tablespoon of garlic-mixed olive oil

- 1 piece of ginger, the size of the thumb, hacked

- 2 entire chicken breasts

- Zest and squeeze of ½ of a lime

- Pinch of salt

- Pinch of bean stew flakes

Directions:

1. Place chicken bosoms on a sheet of stick film.
2. Overlay the stick film over the chicken to cover.

3. Take a moving pin and pound the chicken bosoms level and equally thin.
4. Remove he stick film and discard.
5. Put the chicken in a medium-sized bowl.
6. Take every one of the excess fixings and spot in a blender or food processor.
7. Beat until a smooth glue structures.
8. Add additional water to slacken the glue a bit and hold it back from getting too dry.
9. Add the glue to the chicken. Blend well to cover the chicken equitably.
10. Marinate for somewhere around 2 hours in the refrigerator.
11. Grill or grill the chicken escalopes for around 10 minutes on each side.
12. Transform most of the way into the cooking to get extraordinary barbecue marks.
13. The chicken is done in the event that there are no pink meats anyplace. The juices should likewise run clear.

14. Serve warm with salad, earthy colored rice or sans gluten pita bread.

Breakfast Wrap

Ingredients:

- 1 medium tomato

- Potatoes

- 1-2 slices of low-FODMAP cheese (e.g., cheddar)

- ⅛ of the whole avocado

- ½ cup of spinach

- Scrambled eggs (try only egg whites if you are sensitive to whole eggs)

- ½ cup of bell peppers

- 1 bunch of green onions/scallions (only use green part)

Directions:

1. Select the INGREDIENTS: you would like to include in your wrap and prepare them in any way you would like.

2. For example, you can either roast/sauté your veggies or simply include them raw.

3. Once you have the INGREDIENTS: you like, simply wrap up the cooked tortilla around the filling and you have a wholesome breakfast. Enjoy!

French Toast With Banana And Pecans

Ingredients:

- 1 a banana

- ½ tbsp olive oil spread or dairy-free butter

- 1 tsp of ground cinnamon

- 2 tsp of maple syrup pure

- 2 tbsp of crumbled pecans (OR sunflower/pumpkin seeds)

- 1 large frying pan

- 1 wide, flat bowl

- 1 egg

- 2 slices of a low-FODMAP bread

Directions:

1. Begin to heat your large frying pan over medium heat.

2. As it heats up, add in your dairy-free butter or olive oil spread and let it sit.

3. In your flat, wide bowl, begin to scramble your egg and add in the cinnamon.

4. One slice at a time, place your bread in the egg bowl, and make sure to coat the bread slices completely with the mixture.

5. Give the bread time to soak up the egg fully, so after you have finished dipping both slices, there should be no egg mixture left in the bowl.

6. Now, place the soaked bread in your frying pan, and cook each side of each slice for about 2–3 minutes until you achieve a golden-brown hue.

7. To serve, the French toast, lay the bread on a medium plate while still hot, and top it with sliced bananas and pecan bits (or the toasted sunflower or pumpkin seeds) and drizzle some pure maple syrup over the top. Enjoy!

Florentine Eggs

Ingredients:

- Dash of white vinegar

- 4 fresh eggs, at room temperature

- 4 slices gluten free bread, toasted

- 8 thin bacon slices

- 1 ounce pat of butter

- 2 bunches spinach, trimmed, washed, dried

Hollandaise sauce

- 2 egg yolks

- 7 ounces unsalted butter, melted

- 2 teaspoons lemon juice

- 1/4 cup white wine vinegar

- 6 black peppercorns

Directions:

Begin with the Hollandaise Sauce:

1. Combine the vinegar, peppercorns in a small pan over a low flame. Simmer these INGREDIENTS: for 3-5 minutes, until the liquid is reduced to 2 teaspoons. Remove the pan from the heat and pour the liquid base through a fine colander. Keep the liquid for the hollandaise sauce.

2. Place the vinegar base and the egg yolks into a double boiler, whisking continually. Add the melted better in a slow stream, while whisking to create an even mix. Whisk until the sauce changes texture from thin to thick and creamy. Season with pepper and salt to taste. Add the lemon juice to the sauce and whisk to combine. Set aside and cover with foil as you prepare the eggs and bacon.

3. Heat a frying pan over high heat, add the bacon and fry until crisp. Place on a paper

towel to drain. Melt the remaining butter in the frying pan until the butter foams. Place the spinach into the pan and saute, 4 minutes or so, until the spinach wilts. Salt and pepper to taste.

To Poach the Eggs:

1. Heat a large pan over high heat filled with water. Add a dash of vinegar and reduce the heat to a slow simmer. Crack the egg into a cup, gently so as not to bruise the yolk. Use a wooden spoon to stir the water to ripple like a whirlpool. Gently pour the egg into the whirlpool and cook for 2 minutes for a soft centered egg, or longer if you desire.

2. Using a slotted spoon, transfer the egg onto the plate. Cover with foil to keep warm while cooking the remaining eggs.

3. Place the toast in a pleasing arrangement onto the serving plates.

4. Spoon first the spinach, then the bacon, and then the eggs onto the toast slices.

5. Pour the hollandaise sauce in a small stream over each plate, then garnish with parsley and a small slice of lemon.

6. Serve immediately with salt and pepper.

Frittata With Spinach And Ham

Ingredients:

- 1/2 cup pure cream or lactose free milk

- 1/3 cup grated parmesan cheese

- 250g cherry tomatoes, halved

- 1 bunch spinach, trimmed, shredded

- 100g ham, chopped

- 6 eggs

Directions:

1. Preheat the oven to 375F. Place parchment paper into an 8 x 8 glass pan. Grease the parchment paper and make sure there is a 2 inch overhang on 2 of the sides.

2. Layer half of the spinach into the pan. Top with half of the ham. Continue to layer the

spinach and the ham. There should be four layers total.

3. Mix the eggs, cheese, and milk or milk substitute into a bowl, combining thoroughly. Add salt and pepper and pour over the top of the spinach and ham. Arrange the tomatoes on top, with the cut sides upturned.

4. Bake 35 to 40 minutes until golden brown and the eggs are set. Rest 10 minutes before cutting. Serve with gluten free rolls or toast and a small serving of strawberries or raspberries on the side.

Egg Shakshuka

Ingredients:

- 1/8 teaspoon dried chili flakes

- 2 tablespoons garlic-infused oil

- 2 teaspoons cumin, ground

- 400 grams canned tomatoes, crushed

- 2 teaspoons paprika

- 250 milliliters low FODMAP chicken stock

- 1 red bell pepper

- 8 slices spelt sourdough or wheat bread

- 60 grams baby spinach, chopped roughly

- 4 large eggs

- 2 tablespoons corn starch

- 10 grams green onions

Directions:

1. Prepare the vegetables. Remove the seeds of the red bell pepper and slice it into thick strips.

2. Remove the white stem of the green onions and chop the green tips finely.

3. Over medium heat, cook the bell pepper strips using garlic-infused oil in a frying pan until soft.

4. Pour the chicken stock into the frying pan and add tomatoes. Stir well.

5. Bring the mixture into a simmer and allow to cook for 2 minutes.

6. Place warm water in a bowl and add corn starch. Stir until all of the powder is dissolved then mix it with the sauce in the frying pan.

7. Add green onions and spinach to the sauce. Cook for 2 minutes.

8. Season the sauce with paprika, chili flakes, salt, cumin and pepper. Reduce the heat to medium-low.

9. Crack the eggs and place them in the sauce. Make sure to arrange them evenly around the frying pan.

10. Place a lid on the frying pan and let the contents simmer until the eggs are cooked as desired.

11. Serve the egg shakshuka with bread slices.

Blueberry Smoothie

Ingredients:

- 20 pieces frozen blueberries

- 2 teaspoons chia seeds

- 6 pieces ice cube

- 3 teaspoons rice protein powder

- 30 grams frozen, firm banana, sliced

- 125 milliliters almond milk

- 2 teaspoons lemon juice

- 60 milliliters vanilla soy ice cream

- ½ tablespoon pure maple syrup

Directions:

1. Put all of the INGREDIENTS: in a blender.
2. Blend until a smooth texture is obtained.
3. Consume immediately.

Carrot, Coconut & Ginger Soup

Ingredients:

- 4 tbsp coconut milk

- 1 tbsp apple juice vinegar

- 1 tsp turmeric

- 1 tbsp paprika

- 8 carrots

- 4 parsnips

- 1-inch lump of ginger

- 1-liter bubbling water or FODMAP-accommodating vegetable stock

- Ocean salt and split dark pepper, to taste

- Garnishes of decision, for example, pumpkin or sunflower seeds

Directions:

1. Strip the carrots, parsnips, and ginger and cleave into little pieces.
2. Spot the vegetables and ginger in a container and include the bubbling water.
3. Include the turmeric, paprika, and salt and pepper and permit to stew for 15-20 minutes or until vegetables are delicate.
4. When cooked, enable the blend to cool before moving into a blender.
5. Include the coconut milk and apple juice vinegar and rush until smooth.
6. Fill bowls and top with an additional twirl of coconut milk, a bunch of pumpkin seeds and a bunch of hemp seeds or some other fixings of decision.

Slow Cooker Chicken And Wild Rice Soup

Ingredients:

- 3/4 cup wild rice-dark colored rice mix (I use Lundberg)

- 2 egg yolks (discretionary)

- 2 tsp garlic-implanted or standard olive oil

- 1 little leek, green parts just, cut

- 3 tbsp lemon juice (from 1 lemon)

- Salt and dark pepper to taste

- Ground parmesan cheddar for serving

- Hacked new Italian parsley for serving

- 4 carrots, stripped and cleaved

- 1 huge zucchini, slashed

- 1 lb boneless, skinless chicken bosoms, cut down the middle assuming huge

- 1 tbsp spread

- 1/2 teaspoon dried herbes de Provence or dried thyme

- 1 straight leaf

- 4 cups chicken stock

- 1 cup of water

Directions:

1. Add all fixings through the rice to a huge moderate cooker and cook until chicken bosoms are obscure in the thickest part (165F on a moment read thermometer) and rice is delicate, 4 hours on high, or 8 hours on low. Move chicken bosoms to a cutting board.
2. In a little bowl, whisk the egg yolks.

3. Gradually pour about ¼ cup of the hot soup into the yolks as you whisk (this warms up the yolks, so they don't begin to scramble when you add them to the hot soup).

4. With the moderate cooker on high, gradually empty the yolk blend into the soup, mixing as you pour.

5. Spread the moderate cooker and cook on high for 10 minutes.

6. Warmth the garlic oil in a skillet on medium warmth. Include leek, season with salt and pepper, and cook until delicate, 6 to 8 minutes.

7. Shred the chicken and add it back to the moderate cooker alongside the leeks.

8. Cover and cook for a couple of moments, just until chicken is warmed through.

9. If soup is extremely thick, include water or juices (I included about ½ cup) to thin as you

like. Mood killer moderate cooker and mix in the lemon juice.

10. Season to taste with salt and dark pepper. Scoop into bowls and top with Parmesan and crisp parsley.

Thai-Style Rice And Meat Noodles

Ingredients:

- 1/2 chilli

- 200 g sirloin steak

- 60 g rice noodles

- 115 g broccoli

- ½ carrot, grated

- 45 g soybeans

- 1 tbsp mint, finely chopped

- 1.5 tablespoons of lime juice

- 1 tbsp fish sauce

- 1 tbsp olive oil

- 1 tbsp sugar

- Salt

Directions:

Marinate the meat

1. Pour the lime juice, fish sauce, oil, sugar and chilli into a bowl.
2. Mix everything well.
3. Take 2 tablespoons of this marinade and put them in a bowl and set the rest aside.
4. Arrange the meat and turn it over to sprinkle it well with the marinade.
5. Cover and leave to rest in the refrigerator for an hour.
6. Cook the spaghetti and broccoli
7. Cook the spaghetti al dente in a pot of boiling salted water. Drain them and pour them into a bowl.
8. Cook the broccoli al dente in a pot of boiling salted water. Drain them and put them in the salad bowl.

9. Add the carrot, bean sprouts and mint, season with the reserved marinade and mix.

10. Cook the meat on the barbecue or in a pan and cut into thin slices. Then arrange them in the salad bowl.

Turkey Burger With Cheese

Ingredients:

- 20 g of gorgonzola

- 4 slices of gluten-free bread (180 g)

- 1 teaspoon of olive oil

- 1 teaspoon of ketchup (optional)

- 1 teaspoon of mustard (optional)

- ½ stalk of celery, coarsely chopped (35 g)

- 225 g of turkey or ground chicken

- 1/2 tablespoon of oregano

- 1 teaspoon of mustard

- Salt

- Pepper

Directions:

1. Put the first four ingredients in a bowl. Add salt and pepper as required.
2. Mix first with a fork and then with your hands.
3. Create 4 burgers.
4. Divide the cheese and place it in the center of the hamburger.
5. Overlap the other 2 burgers by pressing on the edges to close the cheese well inside.
6. Cook in a previously oiled pan or grill.
7. After about 5 minutes, turn the burgers and cook for another 5 minutes, until the meat is completely cooked.
8. Insert each hamburger between 2 slices of gluten-free bread.
9. Serve with mustard and ketchup to taste, adding a lettuce leaf and tomato wedge if you like.

Chicken Caesar Salad

Ingredients:

- 1 tablespoon vinegar

- 20 g bacon, diced

- 1/2 romaine lettuce Salt

- Pepper

- 2 tablespoons grated Parmesan

- 300 g of chicken breast

- 3 tablespoons of flavored oil garlic

- 2 chopped anchovy fillets

- 1 yolk

- 1 teaspoon mustard

- 1 teaspoon Tabasco sauce

Directions:

1. You can cook the chicken on the barbecue or on the grill of a preheated oven.
2. Sprinkle the chicken with a little oil, salt and pepper and cook for about ten minutes, turning it halfway through cooking.
3. When it is well cooked and golden, place it on a cutting board and cover with aluminum foil.
4. Pour a tablespoon of garlic flavored oil into a saucepan over low heat.
5. Add the anchovies, stirring with a spoon for a minute until they are dissolved.
6. Put the egg yolks in a bowl, along with the mustard, Tabasco sauce and vinegar. Stir vigorously with a fork and then slowly pour in the garlic flavored oil, whisking until emulsion.
7. Add the oil with the anchovies and season with salt and pepper.

8. Heat the bacon in a non-stick pan. Once browned, place it on absorbent paper to remove some fat.

9. Wash and dry the lettuce and put it in a salad bowl after having cut it up.

10. Incorporate the bacon, season with the sauce and mix well.

11. Cut thin slices of chicken and place them on the salad. Sprinkle with Parmesan and serve.

Orange Barbecue

Ingredients:

- 1 tsp of orange extract

- 2 tbsp of olive oil

- 1 tsp of barbecue seasoning mix

- 1 cup of chopped lettuce

- 1 small red onion, chopped

- 4 large pieces of chicken breast, boneless

- 1 medium onion, chopped

- 2 small chili peppers

- ½ cup of chicken broth

- ¼ cup of fresh orange juice

Directions:

1. Heat up the olive oil in a large saucepan. Add chopped onions and fry for several minutes, over a medium temperature – until golden color.

2. Combine chili peppers, orange juice and orange extract. Mix well in a food processor for 20-30 seconds. Add this mixture into a saucepan and stir well. Reduce heat to simmer.

3. Coat the chicken with barbecue seasoning mix and put into a saucepan. Add chicken broth and bring it to boil. Cook over a medium temperature until the water evaporates. Remove from the heat.

4. Serve with chopped lettuce and red onion.

Chicken Wraps

Ingredients:

- ½ tsp of sea salt

- ¼ tsp of ground pepper

- 4 cups of chopped lettuce

- 1 cup of diced tomato

- ½ cup of onion, sliced

- 1 package of grain-free tortillas

- 1 pound of chicken breast, boneless and skinless

- 2 cups of chicken broth

- 1 cup of lactose-free Greek yogurt

- 1 cup of fresh parsley, chopped

Directions:

1. Combine chicken broth and chicken meat in a sauce pan over medium heat.
2. Cover the sauce pan and allow it to boil.
3. Cook for another 10-15 over medium-low heat. Remove from heat and drain. Let it stand for a while.
4. Chop the meat into bite size pieces.
5. Meanwhile, in a large bowl, combine Greek yogurt, chicken meat, parsley, salt and pepper.
6. Mix gently until the chicken is well coated.
7. Spread this mixture over gluten-free tortillas and top with lettuce, tomato and onion. Roll and serve.

Perfect Scrambled Eggs Recipe

Ingredients:

- 6 tbsp single cream or full cream milk

- A knob of butter

- 2 large free range eggs

Directions:

1. Lightly whisk 2 large eggs, 6 tbsp single cream or full cream milk and a pinch of salt together until the mixture has just one consistency.

2. Heat a small non-stick frying pan for a minute or so, then add a knob of butter and let it melt. Don't allow the butter to brown or it will discolour the eggs.

3. Pour in the egg mixture and let it sit, without stirring, for 20 seconds. Stir with a wooden spoon, lifting and folding it over from the bottom of the pan.

4. Let it sit for another 10 seconds then stir and fold again.

5. Repeat until the eggs are softly set and slightly runny in places. Remove from the heat and leave for a moment to finish cooking.

6. Give a final stir and serve the velvety scramble without delay.

POTATO SALAD WITH ANCHOVY & quail's EGGS

Ingredients:

- 1 anchovy , finely chopped

- 1 tbsp chopped parsley

- 1 tbsp chopped chives

- Juice 0.5 lemon

- 4 quail's eggs

- 100g green beans

- 100g new potatoes , halved or quartered if very large

Directions:

1. Bring a medium pan of water to a simmer. Lower the quail's eggs into the water and cook for 2 mins.

2. Lift out the eggs with a slotted spoon and put into a bowl of cold water.

3. Add the beans to the pan, simmer for 4 mins until tender, then remove from the pan with a slotted spoon and plunge into the bowl of cold water.

4. Put the potatoes in the pan and boil for 10-15 mins until tender.

5. Drain the potatoes in a colander and leave them to cool.

6. While the potatoes are cooling, peel the eggs and cut them in half. Toss the potatoes and beans with the chopped anchovy, herbs and lemon juice. Top with the quail's eggs to serve.

Gluten-Free Carrot Cake

Ingredients:

- 1 tsp cinnamon

- 1 tsp gluten-free baking powder

- 50g mixed nut , chopped

- For the icing

- 75g butter , softened

- 175g icing sugar

- 3 tsp cinnamon , plus extra for dusting

- 140g unsalted butter , softened, plus extra for greasing

- 200g caster sugar

- 250g carrots , grated

- 140g sultanas

- 2 eggs , lightly beaten

- 200g gluten-free self-raising flour

Directions:

1. Heat oven to 180C/160C fan/gas 4. Grease and line a 900g/2lb loaf tin with baking parchment.
2. Beat the butter and sugar until soft and creamy, then stir in the grated carrot and sultanas.
3. Pour the eggs into the mix a little at a time.
4. Add the flour, cinnamon, baking powder and most of the chopped nuts and mix well.
5. Tip the mix into the loaf tin, then bake for 50-55 mins or until a skewer poked in the middle comes out clean.
6. Allow to cool in the tin for 15 mins, then remove from the tin and cool completely on a wire rack.

7. Meanwhile, make the icing. Beat the butter in a large bowl until it is really soft, add the icing sugar and cinnamon, then beat until thick and creamy.

8. When the cake is cool, spread the icing on top, then sprinkle with a little more cinnamon and the remaining chopped nuts.

Gluten-Free Okonomiyaki

Ingredients:

For the pancakes:

- 1/3 cup white rice flour

- 6 cups finely shredded cabbage

- 4 scallions thinly sliced

- Grapeseed or refined coconut oil for frying

- 4 eggs

- 1 teaspoon gluten-free tamari

- 1 teaspoon toasted sesame oil

- 1 teaspoon sea salt plus more for seasoning

For the dipping sauce:

- 1/2 teaspoon hot sauce or Sriracha

- ½ teaspoon toasted sesame oil

- 1/2 teaspoon honey

- 2 tablespoons gluten-free tamari

- 1 tablespoon rice vinegar

- 1 tablespoon mirin

Directions:

1. In a large mixing bowl, whisk together the eggs, tamari, sesame oil, and salt. Fold in the flour until incorporated and all the lumps are out. Stir in cabbage and scallions.

2. In a large heavy skillet (I like cast iron), warm a couple tablespoons of oil over medium-high heat until glistening. Add the cabbage batter in heaping tablespoons to the skillet, frying about 4 at a time. Lower the heat to medium. Cook on each side for about 3 minutes or until golden brown. Transfer to a paper-towel lined plate and season lightly with salt. Repeat with the remaining cabbage, making sure to re-mix

before each round, as the egg tends to fall to the bottom.

3. While the cabbage is frying, make the sauce: combine all ingredients in a small bowl. Add 1 tablespoon of water. Set aside.

4. Serve the pancakes immediately with the sauce on the side. Alternatively, you can make them in advance and recrisp on a baking sheet in a 400-degree oven for 15 minutes before eating.

Vegan Brown Rice Jambalaya With Black Eyed Peas And Collards

Ingredients:

- 1/2 teaspoon ground cumin

- 1/4 teaspoon cayenne

- 2 cups chopped tomatoes or one 15-ounce can diced tomatoes in their juices

- 2 bay leaves

- 4 sprigs fresh thyme

- 8 cups vegetable stock

- 2 cups dried black-eyed peas soaked overnight

- 2 cups American long grain brown rice

- 1 bunch scallions thinly sliced

- 2 tablespoons chopped flat-leaf parsley

- 4 tablespoons olive oil divided

- 1 bunch collard greens thick stems removed and thinly sliced

- Sea salt & pepper

- 1 small yellow onion

- 1 red bell pepper finely diced

- 2 celery stalks thinly sliced

- 1 large jalapeno seeds and ribs removed, minced

- 2 cloves garlic minced

- 1 teaspoon smoked paprika

- 1 teaspoon paprika

Directions:

1. In a large pot over medium-high heat, add 2 tablespoons of the olive oil. Add the collard greens and stir-fry until wilted and tender, about 5 minutes. Season with salt and pepper and remove to a plate. Set aside.

2. Add the remaining olive oil along with the onions, bell pepper, and celery, and sauté until soft, about 5 minutes. Stir in the jalapeno, garlic, smoked paprika, regular paprika, cumin, cayenne, and salt. Cook for 2 minutes more, until very fragrant, then add the tomatoes, bay leaves, and thyme. Bring to a simmer and allow the tomato mixture to thicken slightly.

3. Pour in the stock, black-eyed peas, and brown rice. Bring to a boil, partially cover, and reduce the heat to medium-low. Simmer for 35 minutes, stirring occasionally, until the peas and rice have grown in size, but still have quite a bite to them. Cover the pot

completely and continue cooking over low heat, undisturbed, until tender (but not mushy) and all of the liquid has been absorbed, another 20 minutes.

4. Fold in the collard greens and half the scallions. Cover and cook until the rice has absorbed all the liquid and the veggies are tender, about 10 minutes longer. Remove from the heat.

5. Season the vegetarian jambalaya with parsley, the remaining scallions, and serve warm.

Blender Oat + Pumpkin Muffins

Ingredients:

- 1 teaspoon cinnamon

- 2 large eggs

- 1 teaspoon baking soda

- 3 tablespoons maple syrup

- 1/4 cup olive oil

- 2 1/4 cup old fashioned rolled oats

- 1 cup pumpkin puree

- 1 teaspoon pumpkin spice seasoning

- 1/2 cup lactose free cow's milk (can sub in suitable almond or rice milk)

- Toppings: rolled oats, chia seeds, hemp seeds, pumpkin seeds, dark chocolate chips, chopped pecans

122

Directions:

1. Preheat oven to 350 degrees F.
2. Add oats, pumpkin, pumpkin spice seasoning, cinnamon, eggs, baking soda, maple syrup, olive oil, lactose free milk in to blender.
3. Blend mixture until creamy, about 2 minutes.
4. Add batter to lightly oiled muffin tins, filling muffin cup about 3/4 full.
5. Sprinkle top of muffins with about 1/2-1 teaspoon of the various toppings, as desired.
6. Bake muffins 20 minutes for traditional muffins or 25 minutes for larger size muffin-- or until cake tester comes out clean.

Caprese Spaghetti Squash

Ingredients:

- 4 ounce fresh mozzarella, chopped into bite size pieces

- 20 cherry tomatoes

- 2 tablespoons roasted pepitas, optional

- 1 bunch fresh basil, chopped (about 1/2 cup chopped)

- 1 medium spaghetti squash, cut in half lengthwise, and de-seeded

- 2 tablespoons extra virgin olive oil

- Salt and pepper, to taste

- 1 1/2 cups fody foods low fodmap marinara sauce (or suitable low fodmap pasta sauce)

Directions:

1. Preheat oven to 400 degrees F.
2. Prepare the spaghetti squash, use a fork and lightly pierce holes in back side of squash.
3. Lightly oil the insides of the squash with 1 tablespoon of oil and salt and pepper, to taste.
4. Roast squash (skin side up) for about 40 minutes on small rimmed baking sheet. Cooking time varies depending on the size of the squash. (tip: you should be able to use a small steak knife to cut through the skin of the squash when it is done cooking).
5. While squash is cooking, roast cherry tomatoes.
6. In small baking dish, add tomatoes and remaining 1 tablespoon olive oil, salt and pepper to taste.

7. Add to oven to roast for 10 minutes. Stir tomatoes about 1/2 way through cooking time for even cooking.

8. When squash is done cooking, remove from oven and let it cool slightly, then flip squash over.

9. Using a fork, lightly scape the spaghetti squash strands.

10. Drizzle about 3/4 cup marinara sauce over each 1/2 squash, blending with fork.

11. Remove roasted tomatoes from oven, and place over squash.

12. Top with mozzarella and place squash back into the oven to melt cheese for another 5-10 minutes.

13. Remove squash from oven when cheese is melted. Garnish squash with pepitas (if using) and plenty of fresh basil.

Thai Salmon Cakes

INGREDIENTS:

- Small measure of corn flour, for tidying (For Dipping Sauce)

- 1 little red bean stew, eliminate the seeds and hack finely 45 ml lime juice (from roughly 2 limes) newly pressed 30 ml of Thai fish sauce

- 1 tablespoons of palm sugar

- 1 tablespoon finely hacked mint

- 1 tablespoon finely cleaved coriander

- 300 grams salmon filets, skin and bones

- eliminated, cut into pieces 1 little red stew, seeds eliminated and cleaved finely 11

- 3 tablespoons of vegetable oil

- 2 teaspoons of Thai fish sauce

- A modest bunch of new coriander leaves, slashed finely Zest of 1 lime, grated

- Finely cleaved green highest points of 2 stalks of spring onions

Directions:

1. Put salmon filets in a food processor. Beat for a couple of times to separate the meat.
2. Assuming no food processor is accessible, cut up the filets into tiny, nearly ground-up pieces.
3. Add bean stew, lemon grass, lime zing, and fish sauce into the food processor.
4. Beat a couple of more cycles to join everything.
5. Assuming that no food processor, add these fixings into the cut-up salmon filets and keep hacking until everything is in little pieces.
6. Divide the filet blend into 10 balls.

7. Roll between the hands to form into a ball and afterward smooth into plates about ½-inch thick. Dust each fishcake with a limited quantity of corn flour.

8. This forestalls the fish cakes from turning out to be too sticky.

9. Heat container and add oil. Cook the fishcakes until brilliant brown, around 2 minutes on each side.

10. For the plunging sauce, consolidate all fixings in a little bowl.

11. Serve fishcakes with plunging sauce on the side.

Courgette Pasta With Pine Nuts

Ingredients:

- 5 anchovy fillets

- 1 tablespoon of garlic-implanted olive oil in addition to some extra to complete A little spot of dried bean stew flakes

- Grated parmesan cheese

- 180 grams sans gluten pasta

- 1 medium-sized courgette, cut into short sticks A modest bunch of pine nuts

- A touch of ground dark pepper

Directions:

1. Cook pasta in a huge pot of bubbling water.
2. Cook as indicated by bundle guidelines, until still somewhat firm.

3. Mix sometimes while cooking to keep the pasta from adhering to the base.

4. Channel when cooked however saved 50 ml of the cooking water.

5. Heat skillet over medium hotness settings.

6. Gently toast pine nuts with next to no additional oils.

7. Throw until the nuts begin to brown and become fragrant. Eliminate from the container and set aside.

8. In a similar dish, add garlic-mixed olive oil.

9. Add the anchovy filets advertisement the stew drops.

10. Separate the anchovies with a wooden spoon and fry for a couple minutes.

11. Add courgette and pan fried food until it begins to mellow. Transform off the heat.

12. Add the cooked pasta into the dish. Add saved pasta cooking water and a big part of the parmesan cheddar.

13. Throw to blend all that together.

14. Serve by fixing with pine nuts and remaining parmesan cheddar.

15. Shower a modest quantity of garlic-mixed olive oil.

Tofu Breakfast Scramble

Ingredients:

- ½ cup of grated carrots

- ½ cup of grated zucchini

- 1 tsp of soy sauce

- ¼ tsp of ground turmeric

- 2 tsp of cooking spray (or cooking oil)

- 1 small to a medium mixing bowl

- 1 small to a medium frying pan

- 100 g of medium-firm or firm tofu

Directions:

1. Begin by adding about ¼ cup of water to your mixing bowl.

2. Stir in the soy sauce and ground turmeric, and make sure to mix both well with the water.

3. Take your tofu and use your fingers to crumble it up, piece by piece.

4. Let the bits fall into the mixing bowl and mix them with the water, soy sauce, and ground turmeric.

5. Add in your grated or diced (based on personal preference) carrots and zucchini.

6. Add the cooking oil to your medium frying pan, and set it over a medium flame.

7. Adding oil to this recipe helps give your tofu a yellowish color and will make the scramble look more like scrambled eggs.

8. Once the oil has begun to heat up, add the entire contents of the mixing bowl into the frying pan, and let everything cook through.

9. You will know the tofu is ready when it has a sort of yellow or golden-brown color on all surfaces.

10. Serve the scramble on a plate with a slice of low-FODMAP bread and enjoy!

11. Although personalized Directions:s are not made explicit in this recipe, do feel free to change your tofu scramble by adding in different spices and veggies or by topping your scramble with some type of garnish. You can also swap out the low-FODMAP bread with some low-FODMAP rice.

12. Please make sure that you use this freedom responsibly! Check that everything you buy and the quantities you use for this recipe are all low-FODMAP. Enjoy your customizable tofu scramble!

Salmon Fried Rice

Ingredients:

- ½ cup of finely chopped green onions/scallions (only use green part)

- 2 tbsp of ginger (crushed or grated fresh)

- 210 grams of canned plain pink salmon

- 1 cup uncooked rice (basmati or long-grain white rice)

- OR use 2 cups precooked rice - this option will decrease total cook time

- 1 tbsp of garlic-infused oil

- 1 tbsp of sesame oil

- 2 tbsp of Nam Pla (Thai fish sauce)

- 2 tbsp of soy sauce

- 1 large frying pan

- 1 medium saucepan

- 2 large eggs

- 1 large, peeled, and grated carrot

- 80 grams of green beans

- 1 sliced red bell pepper - deseeded

- Salt and Pepper

Directions:

1. Begin cooking rice in the saucepan according to packet Directions:.
2. Move on to step 2 if you are using precooked rice.
3. Prepare the vegetables as you would like. Suggestions have been included in the ingredient list above.
4. Heat the large frying pan over medium heat and add the garlic-infused oil and sesame oil.

5. Add in the garlic and scallions and cook for not more than 2 minutes until translucent and you can smell the aroma of garlic.
6. Add the slices of bell pepper and sauté for a full minute until softened.
7. Then add green beans, tinned salmon (should be drained from a can), and carrot and stir until salmon breaks into bite-size pieces.
8. At this point, turn the heat down slightly and add in the Thai fish sauce.
9. Crack the eggs into the pan and continually stir all INGREDIENTS: together until the eggs are fully cooked.
10. Add freshly cooked rice to the frying pan and stir in the soy sauce.
11. Season with salt and pepper if desired.
12. Remove from heat once the dish is thoroughly and evenly heated. Plate and enjoy!

Irish Soda Bread

Ingredients:

- 1/2 cup tapioca starch

- 1 1/2 tablespoons powdered dextrose (or 1 tbsp. Sugar)

- 1 teaspoon baking soda

- 1 teaspoon baking powder

- 1/2 teaspoon salt

- Scant 1 cup milk or non-dairy substitute

- 1 tablespoon vinegar or lemon juice

- 1 large egg, lightly beaten

- 1 tablespoon grapeseed oil, light olive oil or canola oil

- 1 1/2 cups white rice flour

Directions:

1. Preheat oven to 350 degrees F. Grease and flour a 9" cake pan or a 9" x 5" loaf pan.

2. Place the 1 T vinegar or lemon juice into a glass measuring cup.

3. Pour enough milk into the measuring cup to equal 1 cup total. Stir the two INGREDIENTS: and let sit for 2 minutes.

4. Combine the milk mix, the egg and the oil into a medium sized bowl.

5. In a larger bowl, place the rice flour, tapioca starch, sugar or dextrose, baking powder, baking soda and salt.

6. Mix these together and then add the milk mixture and stir well with a wooden spoon.

7. Pour into the baking pan and bake for 20-25 minutes until golden brown. Insert a knife into the center to check for doneness.

8. Cool in the pan for 15 minutes then turn onto a plate and serve warm.

Oatmeal With Cinnamon Spiced Bananas

Ingredients:

- 125g brown sugar

- 300ml thickened cream or almond milk

- 2 bananas, sliced

- 4 cups plus 2 T water

- 2 cups (180g) rolled oats (not instant)

- 1/4 teaspoon ground cinnamon, plus extra to dust

Directions:

1. Cook the oats by placing the oats, cinnamon, 4 cups of water and a pinch of salt into a saucepan over medium heat.

2. Bring the oats to a boil and simmer for 3 minutes.

3. Place the sugar in a separate saucepan with 2 T of water.

4. Stir continuously over low heat until the sugar dissolves.

5. Turn up the heat to medium and cook for 2 or 3 minutes until the sugar has carmelized.

6. Add 2/3 of the cream or almond milk and stir over low heat, until a caramel sauce is made.

7. Divide the oat porridge into 6 servings. Place the sliced bananas into the caramel sauce and bathe them.

8. Place them on top of the porridge, sprinkle all with cinnamon, and drizzle with the remaining caramel sauce and milk or cream.

Parmesan, Poppy Seed & Caraway Twists

Ingredients:

- 1 egg , beaten

- 3 tbsp freshly grated parmesan (or vegetarian alternative)

- 1 tbsp each poppy seeds and caraway seeds

- 175g gluten-free flour (we used Doves Farm, widely available)

- 85g butter

- pinch cayenne pepper

- 1 egg yolk mixed with 3 tbsp cold water

Directions:

1. To make the pastry, put the flour, butter and cayenne pepper into a food processor, then whizz into fine breadcrumbs. sprinkle the egg and water mixture onto the flour, then pulse again until the mixture begins to come together. tip the mixture onto a board and gently squeeze the pastry until it begins to come together in a ball, adding more water if it feels dry.

2. Heat oven to 190C/fan 170C/gas 5. roll the pastry into a large a4-sized rectangle, roughly 20 x 30cm.

3. Brush the sheet with the beaten egg and cut in half widthways.

4. Sprinkle one half with the Parmesan and the second half with poppy and caraway seeds. lightly run the rolling pin across the top to press the cheese and the seeds into the pastry.

5. Cut each half into 12-15 sticks. arrange on a baking sheet and chill for 10 mins.

6. Bake for 8-10 mins until golden brown, then cool for 5 mins before lifting onto a wire rack.

Roast Salmon With Preserved Lemon

Ingredients:

- 50g sea salt

- 50g golden caster sugar

- 1 tsp thyme leaves

- 1 tsp chilli flakes

- ½ small bunch dill , washed

- For the preserved lemon roasting oil

- 30g preserved lemons , seeds removed

- 40g preserved lemon , flesh and pith removed

- 100ml gin

- 1kg side organic farmed or wild salmon (tail end)

- 4 tbsp olive oil

Directions:

1. In a food processor, blitz together the lemon and gin.
2. Lay your salmon skin-side down in a roasting tin and pour over the lemon and gin mix.
3. Combine the salt, sugar, thyme and chilli flakes, then spoon over the salmon.
4. Cover with cling film and chill for at least 2 hrs.
5. Heat oven to 160C/140C fan/gas 3. Thirty mins before you want to cook the salmon, remove it from the fridge and allow it to come to room temperature.
6. To make the roasting oil, blitz the preserved lemons and olive oil.
7. Gently rinse the cure from the salmon and pat dry with kitchen paper. Lay it skin-side down in an oiled roasting tray and pour over the roasting oil, rubbing it all over the fish. Cover the tin tightly with foil and roast for 15 mins.

8. Remove the foil and return the fish to the oven for a further 10 mins.

9. Take out of the oven and rest for 5 mins, then scatter over freshly torn dill, to serve.

Vegan Nam Khao

Ingredients:

- 1 1/2 cups jasmine rice or other long grain white rice

- 4 tablespoons coconut oil

- red bell pepper diced

- 1 Fresno chili or jalapeno ribs and seeds removed, minced

- shallot thinly sliced

- 1 tablespoon minced fresh ginger

- bunch lacinato kale stems removed and finely chopped

- teaspoons olive oil

- tablespoons lime juice

- 1/2 teaspoon sea salt

- 1/4 cup gluten-free tamari

- tablespoon rice vinegar

- tablespoon toasted sesame oil

- scallions thinly sliced

- 1/2 cup roughly chopped cilantro

- 1/4 cup roughly chopped peanuts

- 1 lime quartered, for serving

Directions:

1. Place the uncooked rice in a fine mesh strainer and rinse well multiple times. Bring a pot of salted water to a boil and add the rice. Cook the rice for 5 minutes. Drain the rice in the strainer (it will be slightly undercooked and that is okay!) and transfer to a large mixing bowl.

2. In a large lidded skillet or saucepan, heat 2 tablespoons of the coconut oil over a

medium-high flame. Sauté the peppers and shallots until softened, about 5 minutes. Add in the ginger and cook for 1 minute more. Transfer the pepper mixture to the bowl with the rice and toss to combine.

3. Place the skillet back over medium-high heat and add the remaining oil. Once hot, add the rice mixture and use a spatula to press it into one layer, like a rice cake. Wrap the pan lid tightly in a large kitchen towel – be very careful it's not touching the pan or it might char. Cover with the towel-wrapped lid and cook until the rice is golden and crispy, about 7 minutes. Using a flat spatula, flip a few parts of the rice cake and crisp the other side, another 5 minutes. Remove the skillet from the heat, keep it covered with the lid and let it sit for 10 minutes.

4. Meanwhile, in the large mixing bowl, toss the kale with the olive oil, lime juice and salt.

Massage with your hands until dark green and wilted. Set aside.

5. In a small bowl, whisk together the tamari, vinegar and sesame oil.

6. Off the heat, gently toss the crispy rice with the kale and transfer to a serving platter. Drizzle with the tamari mixture. Top with the scallions, cilantro, peanuts and lime wedges.